Alex wilson

Fitness Challenges For Every Age

*Making the Most of Your Body for
the Rest of Your Life*

TABLE

OF CONTENTS

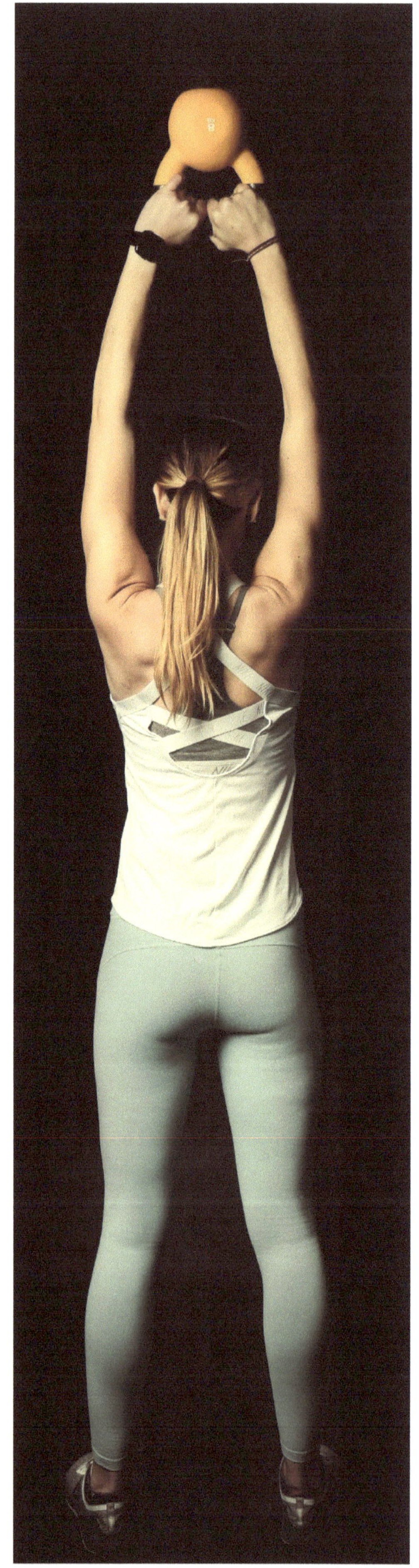

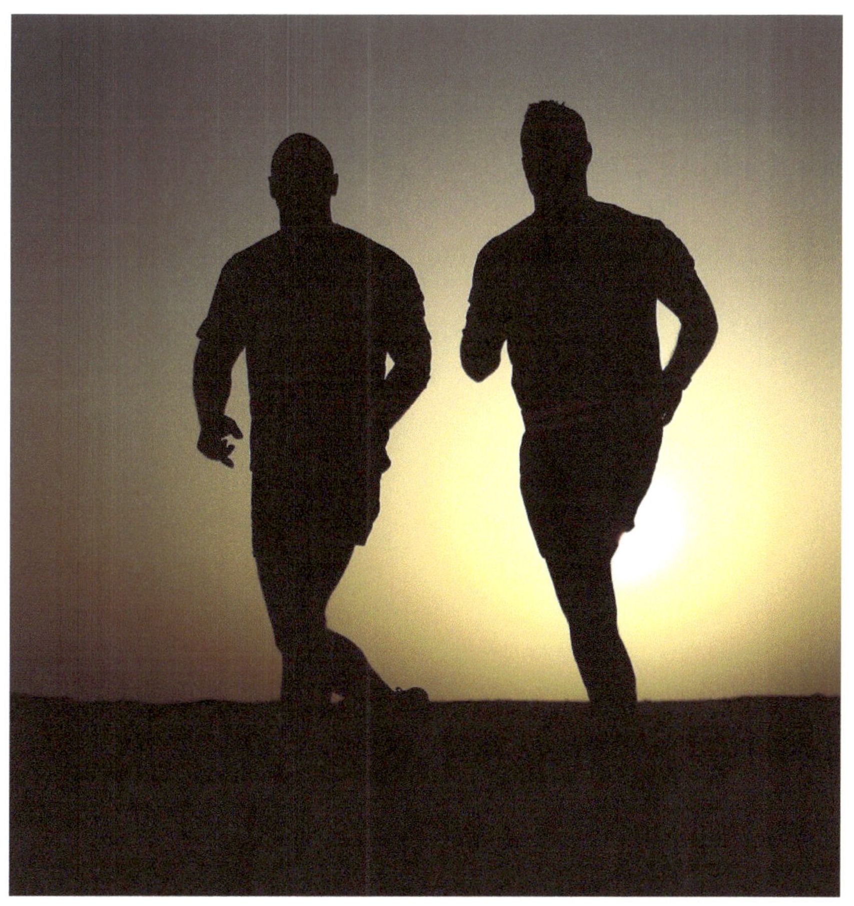

This book is designed for those who want to get started as soon as possible but has no clear and specific idea how. This is obviously the best option for them because all information about nutrition and resistance training is learned through this book. This is the foundation one needs in order to get started and get tips that will last your body for life.

fitness and age

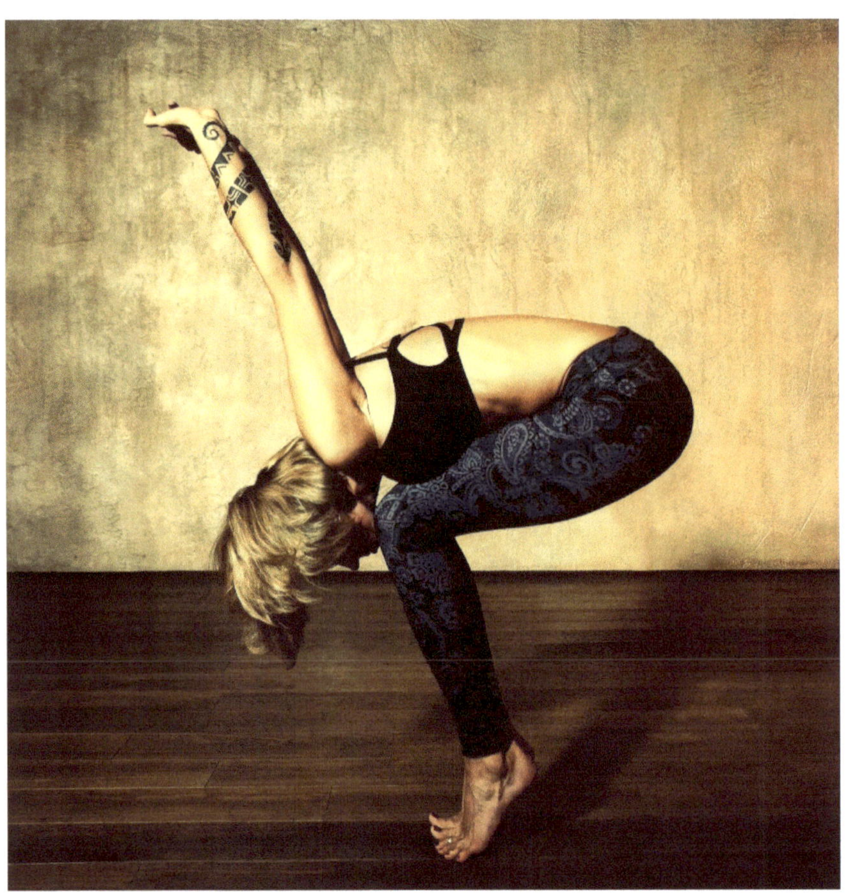

As you develop old, it doesn't imply that you don't have to do wellness works out. Truth be told, you need them like never before. Along these lines, your body will remain physically fit and battle certain medical issues which elderly individuals are progressively inclined to having.

The physical body changes as an individual develops old, and there's no uncertainty about that. Numerous elderly individuals are gradually understanding that and the majority of them can only with significant effort acknowledge such certainty. Changes identified with a person's age is regularly initiated, reversible, and unavoidable. That is a reality that elderly folks individuals ought to acknowledge and manage.

Chapter 2

Beauty and Fitness

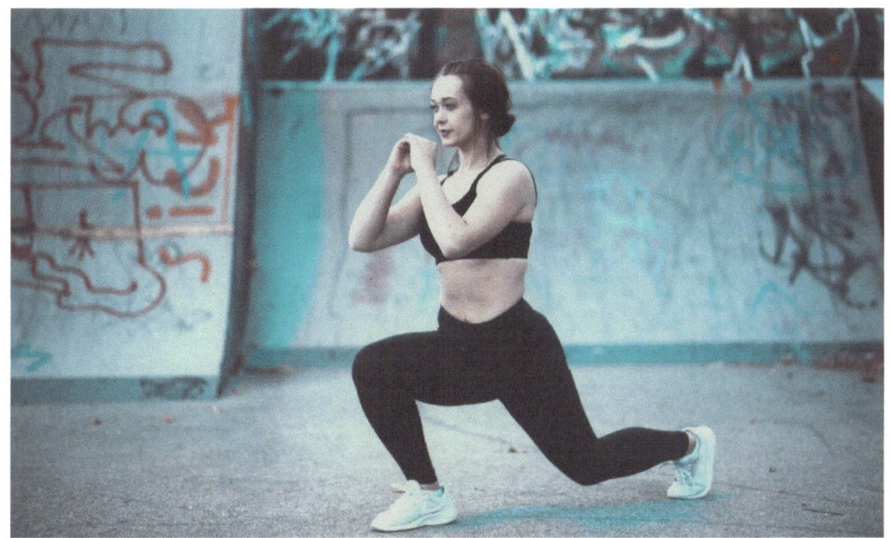

Wellbeing is riches. By being physically fit, it can make an individual look lean both all around.

There is a great deal an individual can do such running or strolling in the first part of the day, playing ball or some other game with companions however on the off chance that an individual needs to have muscles and look fit, the best activity will be to join and exercise in a rec center.

Much the same as taking any drug, one should initially counsel the specialist before experiencing any type of activity.

Physical exercise is useful on the grounds that it keeps up and improve ones wellbeing from an assortment of maladies and unexpected passing. It likewise makes an individual vibe more joyful and builds ones confidence keeping one from falling into sadness or tension. It has likewise appeared to make an individual with a functioning way of life live longer than an individual who doesn't.

The best exercise plan ought to have cardiovascular and weight preparing works out. This helps consume calories and increment the muscle to fat proportion that will build ones digestion and make one either put on or get in shape.

An individual who has never worked out ought to do it steadily. Doing it a lot just because can make one draw a muscle or have damage aggravating it. Continuance will never be worked in a day and doing it over and over will clearly regard the individual.

Concentrating on certain bit in the body can help cause it to improve. A genuine model is setting off to the rec center and doing an exercise all the more regularly in a particular region, for example, the abs can give one a chest pack.

However, magnificence isn't just about having muscles which is the thing that individuals can see. It is likewise about upgrading the excellence inside.

Chapter 3

Moderate Exercises to Fitness

Have you at any point understood worn out and worried from work and when you return home you see your three kids running towards you requesting that you play b-ball with them? You can't and guaranteed them that you will after you take you rest.

Rather than baffling your kids, why not state, "yes" all things considered? You will be shocked by the measure of vitality you will have after that 30-minute movement.

Did you realize that by practicing at a moderate pace for just 30 minutes, you would feel much better, rationally? It has been demonstrated this improves the hunger and hones your style in critical thinking. Not just that. You will likewise feel that it is simpler to rest around evening time in the event that you do direct activities in any event, for just 30 minutes consistently.

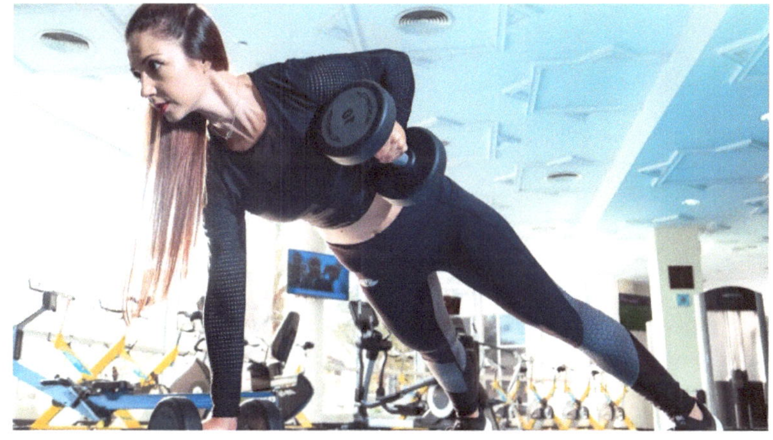

What are the advantages of standard exercise? It advances self-control and has a positive effect how you see life. Exercise helps in lifting your spirits and getting you out of any downturn. For amateurs, it very well may be accomplished for 15 minutes for 2 to 3 days per week. You can expand the time you spend once your body gets adjusted for it.

DON'T you ever drive your body! In the event that you get injured, at that point stop. You can enjoy a reprieve from practicing for a couple of days and after that you can begin again yet you have to begin from day 1.

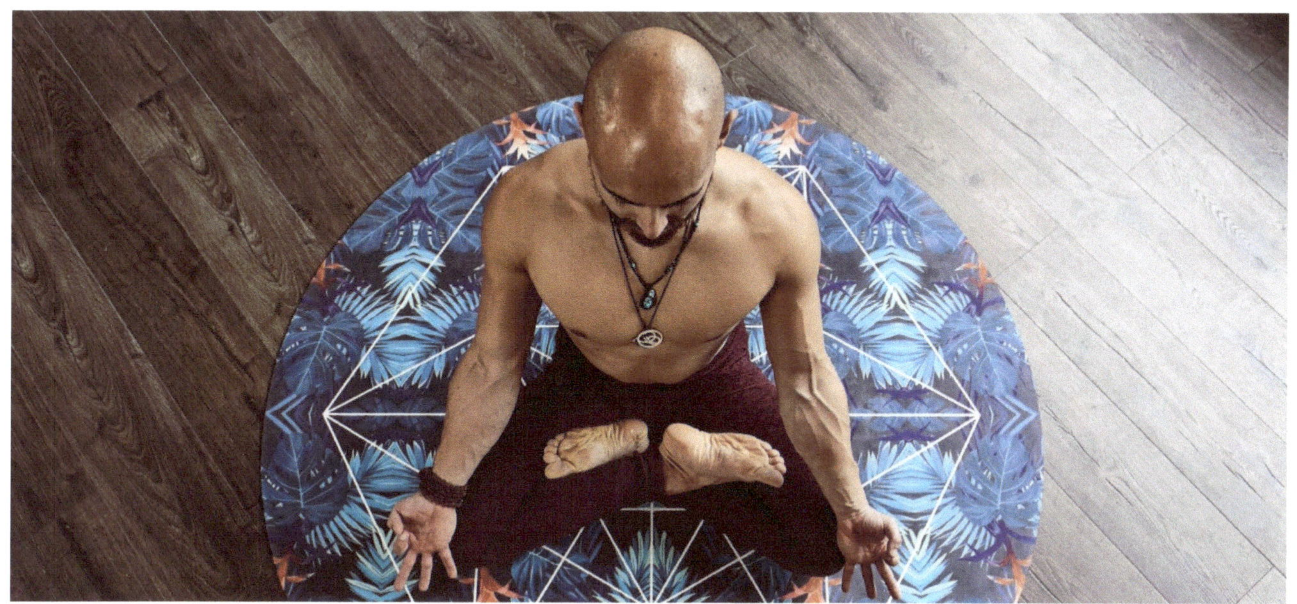

Here are some moderate activities you can do and appreciate:

1. Do the Walking. Utilize your environment. You can walk your canine, with your accomplice or kid. Urge your family to do the strolling exercise day by day and you will end up consuming calories while appreciating the environment and getting enough daylight that is additionally useful for your body.

. 2. Find the marvels of Yoga. Yoga is one viable exercise that stimulates your body as well as your spirit. You might need to adapt even the essential yoga places that are not very convoluted however demonstrated powerful. A five-minute yoga exercise can liven you up and revive your body with the vitality you lost for the entire day. You unwind and simultaneously you stretch!

3. Draw in yourself into sports. Play ball, football, baseball, tennis or badminton. Numerous specialists have prescribed games as a powerful method to remain fit and solid. Sports should likewise be possible with some restraint. Try not to pay attention to it. Shooting ball with a companion is one moderate exercise that is likewise viewed as a game.

4. Join exercise programs at work. On the off chance that despite everything you don't have activities programs at work, at that point why not begin it? You can converse with your manager about it and start with your associates. You don't just lose calories yet it is likewise one great approach to bond with them. This should be possible 30 minutes, 3 times each week.

5. Exercise while doing family unit tasks. Planting, raking leaves, yard cutting, doing the clothing, vacuuming and vehicle washing are viable moderate activities at home. Utilize these errands to perspire and consume calories. Rather than utilizing machines and contraptions to play out these tasks, why not do it with your hands and lose a few fats?

Perhaps the greatest impediment to remaining on track for wellness is losing inspiration. Individuals are simply beginning an activity program can end up immediately tired of a similar daily schedule. Keeping activity engaging and keeping up a decent wellness point of view is vital to long haul achievement.

In the event that you need to watch precisely the same scene of your preferred network show each day for a mind-blowing remainder, you would most likely be slamming your head against the divider before the week's over. You would change the channel, get a book, or do anything you could to abstain from something you once delighted in.

However, numerous individuals beginning a work out schedule feel constrained to pursue a similar everyday practice, for a long time after day, and thus tumble off the activity wagon because of sheer fatigue.

.

That is the reason, the vast majority would need the administrations of a wellness coach so as to give them the various bits of the work out schedule in an increasingly livelier style.

Wellness coaches are really the individuals who are master in examining and making a work out regime that is directly for you. They are the ones who will compute your propriety to a specific program with respect to your "wellness level," make the program as indicated by your particular needs, and keep you animated and enlivened by giving you exercises that won't bore you.

Be that as it may, of course, likewise with different elements incorporated into the wellness world, not all wellness coaches are made equivalent. They may shift from the various trainings that they have, the wellbeing instruction they have gained, and the abilities that they have learned

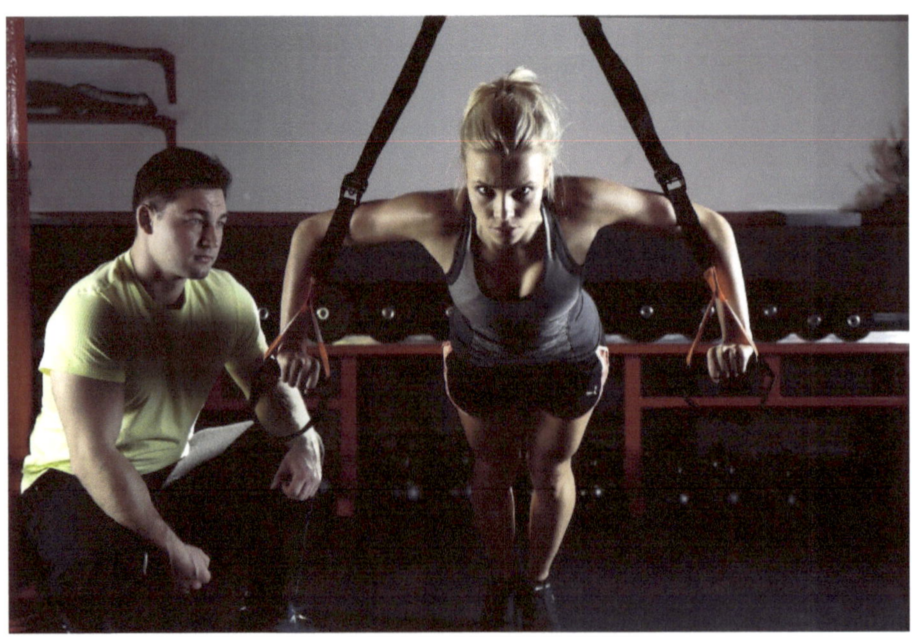

1. Confirmation

Like any thing or item, the quality is now and again estimated and decided through the affirmation that goes with it. Thus, before you pick your wellness coach, it is imperative to check if the mentor is appropriately ensured by an exceptionally respected wellness affiliation.

2. Instruction/Trainings

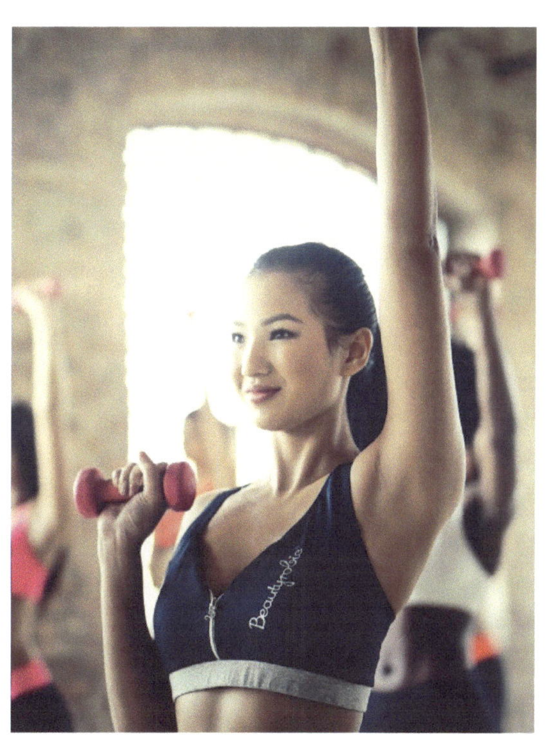

Make certain to pick a wellness coach who had obtained a sufficient preparing and training the extent that wellbeing and physical wellness is concerned. Despite the fact that it isn't fundamental, coaches who have obtained instruction associated with wellbeing or some other related field will have an edge over the others.

3. Realizes how to give the correct consideration

A decent wellness mentor should realize how to give their customer a full focus at whatever point their session is going on. Along these lines, the mentor will have the option to concentrate more on the subtleties that necessities consideration and prompt contemplations.

4. Realizes how to follow advancement

It is ideal to pick a wellness mentor that realizes how to follow their customer's advancement to the extent wellness is concerned.

Along these lines, the coach will have the option to produce new exercises and trainings assigned for a specific aftereffect of the customer.

5. Great Personality

Since you will manage your wellness coach, it is ideal on the off chance that you will search for someone with a satisfying character, someone whom you can be agreeable. It is ideal to contract the administrations of someone whom you can without much of a stretch coexist with.

Come down, the administrations of a wellness focus and the commitments it can give you while working out on those paunch fats, are, in reality, outstanding amongst other assistance that you can get from an expert individual who comprehends what he is doing.

Henceforth, it is ideal to pick the best individual who can give you the best administrations that you need so you will never get exhausted again.

Chapter 4

Diet fitness

Numerous individuals these days are especially cognizant about their very own wellbeing and wellness. Notwithstanding that, these individuals, and numerous others too, are presently wanting to shape their bodies to ahieve that magazine-spread look. Subsequently, exercise centers, wellbeing spas and different wellness focuses have multiplied all over to take into account the necessities of the wellness buffs and fans.

Indeed, even on TV exercise machines, weight reduction items, and other stuff to improve wellness have pretty much overseen the wireless transmissions and advanced into the family units. Be that as it may, exerise isn't the best way to fabricate that body lovely. It likewise involves certain measure of obligation on the nourishments one eats. Being sound and fit expects one to watch diet wellness.

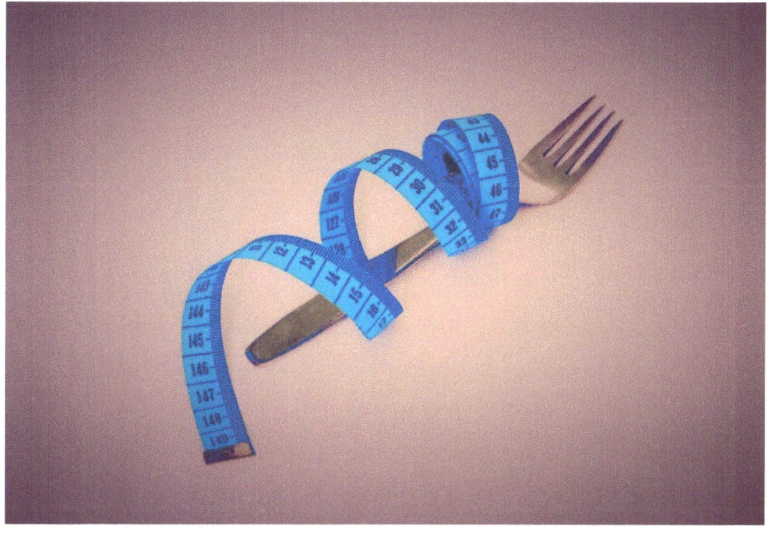

Diet wellness is as basic as exercise itself. Diet for wellness gives the fundamental sustenance one needs to reestablish destroyed muscles and for sound development. Diet wellness ought to never be underestimated. With the fame of staying in shape, a wide range of perspectives, techniques, projects and abstaining from excessive food intake procedures have been defined by numerous experts. Among these are high carb diets and high fat eating regimens. Whih one is progressively successful and which one would it be advisable for one to pursue?

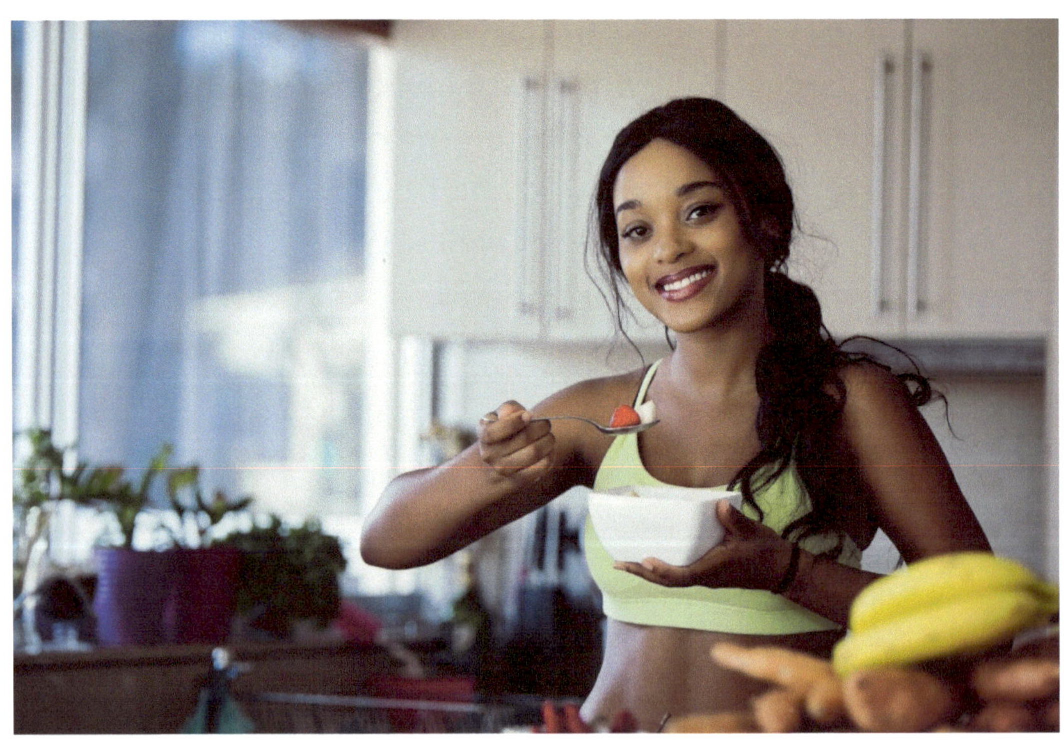

First thing to know would be the central contrasts between these two eating routine approaches. As the name suggests, high carb diets focuses on taking in starch rich nourishments while high fat weight control plans embraces fat-rich food sources. High carb diets are used to glycogen put away in the liver and muscles. Glycogen is a glucose complex that gives a lot of vitality prepared for use in anaerobic activities.

Fats, then again, is well-nown for being the most extravagant wellspring of calories. It really contains 2.5 occasions a larger number of calories than starches and proteins the same. Concentrates additionally show that it takes the body 24 calories to use sugars while it just brings 3 to torch fat. So which one to pursue? An individual can pursue a high carb and low fat wellness diet or the a different way. It is in no way, shape or form prescribed to pursue both simultaneously; except if obviously in the event that you need to pick up muscle versus fat.

In any case, at that point diet wellness isn't tied in with losing fat, one should likewise consider his eating routine so as to ward off fat. Research shows that practical loss of weight must be accomplished on an eating routine which suits the individual nourishment inclinations, way of life, therapeutic profile and satiety signals.

Diet programs all over can assist you with shedding off overabundance pounds, yet just one eating routine can assist you with remaining attractive, and the one fulfills you most. Other significant parts of having a fit eating regimen are control, parity and variety. One must be mindful so as not to forget about significant supplements and different substances fundamental for sound body working. wellbeing associations are clear about the measures of supplements an individual ought to have in the body.

Low fat high carbs, high carbs low fat; the inquiry isn't which diet program will work out yet which is it that will work for you. Taking a stab at a provocative and solid body doesn't need to trouble an individual, diet wellness doesn't need to mean adhering to a similar sort of nourishment forever. One may even attempt to be gutsy and evaluate new nourishments out there. Who knows? one may considerably find spinach intriguing.

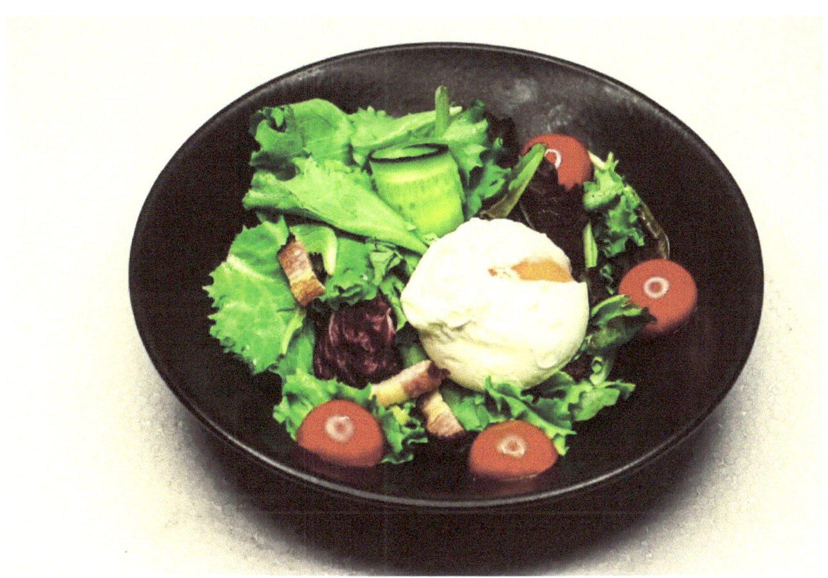

Chapter 5

Home Fitness Gym

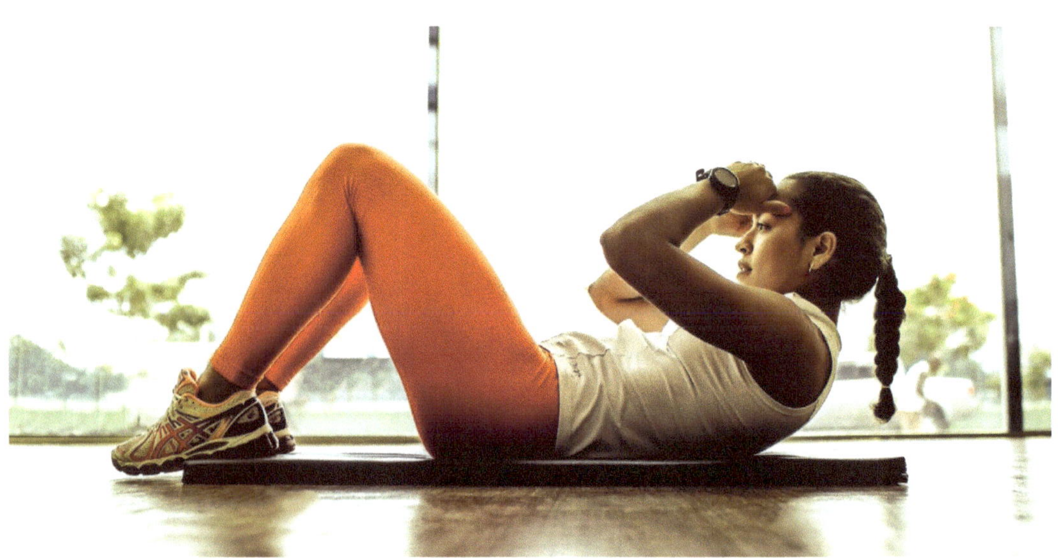

Today, an ever increasing number of individuals are getting to be aware of their figure. But since their so bustling maintaining their lives and their organizations, they don't possess the energy for exercises. Albeit nearby rec center enrollment is truly available and gives all the required types of gear to exercises, still clashes emerge. It can incorporate changing in accordance with the exercise center's opening occasions, worry of making a trip from your home to the rec center, and weight on the climate condition.

In the event that you are confronting this trouble, think about building your own home exercise center to accomplish your wellness objectives and keep you fit as a fiddle. There are different scopes of activity types of gear you can use at home. Time and climate condition isn't an issue any longer. You can do your activities inside your own set timetable. Be that as it may, the inquiry is the thing that types of gear you are going to purchase.

In the event that you are beginning your endeavor, or getting to be dynamic again after a long break, it is prudent not to seek after your home exercise center. Rather you should select at a neighborhood rec center inside a brief timeframe. It can assist you with looking at various wellness types of gear accessible in the market today. You can get some information about its preferences and drawbacks and how these supplies can meet your wellness needs. Consequently, you can rundown down the supplies that you will buy for your home rec center.

You can consider weight machines in the event that you need to exercise explicit gatherings of muscles including the biceps, deltoids, and quadriceps in a more secure way. Progressively finished, free loads can't give great exercises to hamstrings and calves muscle gatherings. Be that as it may, you have to pay the cost of a weight machine. Expenses and setups may broadly fluctuate from a basic obstruction machine, to a customizable, multi-positioned weight stack. You can burn through hundreds or thousands of dollars.

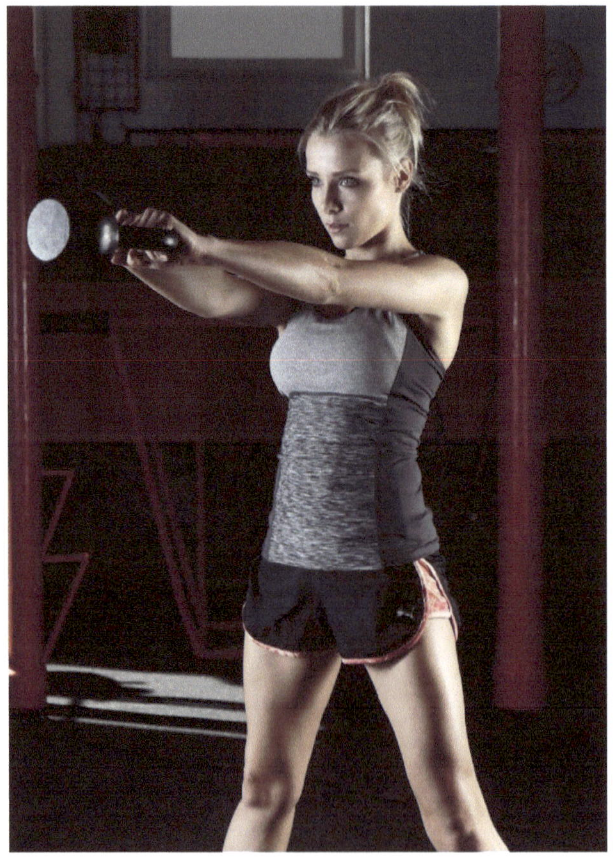

A stair stepper is another prevalent other option. A straightforward stair stepper model can offer you a superior cardiovascular exercise and low effects on your joints when practicing to manufacture your calves and thighs. This machine is likewise a space saver and can cost from 80 to 150 dollars. A progressively unpredictable stair stepper has movable speed, opposition level, speed, pedal separations and that's only the tip of the iceberg. It additionally incorporates a HRM (pulse screen) just as advanced readouts for separation climbed, calories consumed, and speed. It can cost 1,700 to 2,000 dollars. Treadmills are great exercises machines too for your home rec center. The costs rely upon the sorts, models, brand, and highlights.

Building your home rec center can cost you cash. Be that as it may, it merits contributing for to meet your wellness needs.

imprint

Date of Publication

2019

all rights reserved

dedication

I want to thank all
of the readers of
this book .

Alex
wilson